Nuno Miguel Oliveira Ferreira
Ana I.de Almeida R. F. da Rocha
Sofia Marques Grilo Ferreira

Protecting the integuments: Wounds

Nuno Miguel Oliveira Ferreira
Ana I.de Almeida R. F. da Rocha
Sofia Marques Grilo Ferreira

Protecting the integuments: Wounds

Pedagogical Manual

ScienciaScripts

Imprint
Any brand names and product names mentioned in this book are subject to trademark, brand or patent protection and are trademarks or registered trademarks of their respective holders. The use of brand names, product names, common names, trade names, product descriptions etc. even without a particular marking in this work is in no way to be construed to mean that such names may be regarded as unrestricted in respect of trademark and brand protection legislation and could thus be used by anyone.

Cover image: www.ingimage.com

This book is a translation from the original published under ISBN 978-620-6-76019-1.

Publisher:
Sciencia Scripts
is a trademark of
Dodo Books Indian Ocean Ltd. and OmniScriptum S.R.L publishing group

120 High Road, East Finchley, London, N2 9ED, United Kingdom
Str. Armeneasca 28/1, office 1, Chisinau MD-2012, Republic of Moldova, Europe
Printed at: see last page
ISBN: 978-620-7-57921-1

NUNO MIGUEL OLIVEIRA FERREIRA

ANA ISABEL DE ALMEIDA RIBEIRO FERNANDES DA ROCHA

SOFIA MARQUES GRILO FERREIRA

PROTECTING THE INTEGUMENTS: WOUNDS TEACHING MANUAL

PEDAGOGICAL HANDBOOK FOR NURSING STUDENTS,

PRODUCED BY: NUNO FERREIRA; ANA RIBEIRO AND SOFIA FERREIRA

2024

Wounds heal, although they pulsate inside the skin... they are there covered by a layer of skin that has tried to annul them, but they remain there. Wounds are the marks of life that insist on always remaining!!! It's not easy to go on without realising them... they're there... it's not easy to remain without touching them, they're here today and now, pulsating as if it were yesterday in childhood. However, it is possible to learn from them and live with them and make them stop hurting, or to be more humble, to get used to the pain...

Eduardo de Campos Garcia

INDICE

INTRODUCTION

Wound care is complex and requires knowledge and a set of clinical skills in order to promote optimal wound healing and reduce the impact of chronic wounds on the health economy. Nursing students need tools and training to facilitate the care process. It is essential that the approach to the person with a wound is comprehensive, systematic and based on scientific evidence.

Although tissue recovery is a systemic process, it is extremely important to treat the wound site properly in order to facilitate the physiological process.

0 local treatment of wounds is based on scientific studies into the physiology of tissue repair, which is why treatment by technically trained people should always be encouraged. Caring for wounds is a dynamic and complex process in which the nursing student must have a broad vision and play a fundamental role in their treatment. The treatment of wounds is not only "curative", but its main objective is to improve the quality of life of users.

The aim of this pedagogical manual is not only to share experiences, but also to complement knowledge and provide students with the necessary means to apply this knowledge to the reality of their context in the different areas of care:

• Developing basic knowledge in this area and providing contact with new techniques and different ways of working;
• Self-promotion of the ability to make decisions, take initiative, communicate and co-operate, responding to specific situations in the area of wound care with competence and flexibility.
• Indicate and identify the different stages of healing;

• Establish a care plan;

• Select the right dressing material for each type of wound and stage of healing;

• Use the wound bed preparation technique appropriate to the characteristics and tissues of the wound.

1. A HISTORICAL PERSPECTIVE ON WOUND CARE

One of man's main concerns has always been to maintain his health, and wound care is part of this. Since prehistoric times, there has been a great deal of evidence to support this idea, particularly through the observation of drawings, paintings and sculptures on stone.

The first written records date back to around 2500 BC, to clay tablets containing cuneiform writing on which the three healing gestures are described for the first time: washing, plastering and bandaging the wound (Cohen et al. 1998).

What we now call "dressing material", with absorbent and protective properties, were called "plasters" by their ancestors. They were made from various substances, including clay, mud, plants and herbs, and as an adjunct, rose oil and olive oil, a substance associated with religious rituals (Cohen et al. 1998).

It wasn't until the 5th century BC, with Hippocrates (460-375 BC) that medicine emerged as a science based on the natural interpretation of disease. Eternalised in his treatise "On Wounds", which suggested the importance of suppurating wounds in order for them to heal, the concept known as "pus bonum et laudabile" (theory of praiseworthy pus) would later be reaffirmed in a new writing, "On Head Wounds", and remained in force for a long time, greatly influencing Galen and other historic surgeons until the 19th century (Aldini, Fini, & Giardino, 2008).

The great revolution in wound treatment methods came in 1962 with George Winter, and in 1963 with Hinman and Maibach, who demonstrated that healing in a moist environment was more effective than in a dry environment. According to Winter, wounds healed twice as quickly if they were kept in a moist environment (Cohen et al. 1998).

There are currently thousands of products for wound care that are classified as dressings, which must be selected and evaluated in relation to their indications, contraindications, costs and effectiveness.

0technological and scientific development is a daily occurrence, there is an increase in scientific research in the area of wounds and, at the same time, the pharmaceutical industry is making more and more products available. more materials and new technologies for better management of the healing process.

However, the three ancestral steps remain: washing, cleaning and dressing (Cohen et al. 1998), with the aim of preventing infection, protecting and promoting healing. In other words, they are divided into three main stages: assessment, cleaning and selecting the ideal therapeutic option (Alves & Vieira, 2009). Since historical research can help us reflect on the past and the present, it is important to continue reflecting on the developments that have taken place.

2. SKIN ANATOMY AND PHYSIOLOGY

The skin covers the entire surface of the body and is its largest organ. It continues with the mucous membranes that line the digestive, respiratory and urogenital systems where they open onto the surface. It is divided into two distinct layers, the epidermis and dermis, which are firmly attached to each other.

The epidermis is the outermost layer, made up of three different cell lineages: keratin6cytes, melan6cytes and Langerhans cells.

The dermis is the deepest layer and is made up of connective tissue.

The epidermis is organised into layers and, as the more superficial layers are eliminated, the deeper layers are restored by cell division.

It is made up of five layers: Germinal; Spinous; Granular, translucent; C6rnea.

The germ layer is the deepest and borders the dermis.

The horny layer is the most superficial and is made up of squamous cells filled with keratin, providing protection against physical and chemical trauma. The various layers of keratin6cells closely attached to each other provide a barrier against the invasion of microorganisms and water. 0 melanin pigment in the epidermis protects the underlying tissues from the harmful effects of ultraviolet light.

The dermis is a thick layer of connective tissue that extends from the epidermis to the subcutaneous tissue. This layer contains the skin's appendages, many blood vessels, lymphatic vessels and nerves. It can be divided into the papillary layer, which is more external, and the reticular layer, which is more internal. It contains many different cell types, including fibroblasts and fibr6cites, macrophages, mast6cites and blood leuc6cites, particularly neutrophils, eosin6phils, lymph6cites and mon6cites. This layer provides a firm base for the epidermis and skin appendages. The collagen fibres provide great tensile strength and the elastic fibres give the skin flexibility. The vascular plexuses supply blood to the epidermis, without piercing it. The control carried out by the hypothalamus and the sympathetic nerve fibres on the blood flow in the dermis provide a thermoregulation mechanism. The sensory nerve endings in the dermis keep the individual in contact with the environment.

3. WOUND HEALING

Wound healing is subject to a physiological process that comprises several complex cellular steps to restore damaged tissue.

All tissues are capable of self-healing and have two mechanisms for this:

• **Regeneration**: a process in which damaged tissue is replaced by identical cells. In humans, complete regeneration is only possible in some cells, such as liver epithelial cells;

• **Repair**: the process in which damaged tissue is replaced by connective tissue, giving rise to a scar. In humans, it is the main mechanism by which healing occurs.

We can classify wounds according to their etiology, causative agents or healing time. A classic and commonly accepted classification refers to healing time.

Wound healing can be defined as the physiological process by which the body restores and re-establishes the functions of injured tissues.

According to the healing process, wounds are classified as acute or chronic.

Acute wounds are wounds that persist for up to 14 days after surgical intervention or trauma (lacerations, crush injuries, burns). A chronic wound that has been intervened on, for example by debridement, should be considered acute and managed as such.

Chronic wounds are wounds that continue to require treatment after six weeks. Examples are leg ulcers (arterial, venous, phlebitis, cellulitis, neoplastic, neuropathic), pressure ulcers, traumatic wounds, surgical wounds and neoplastic wounds.

3.1. SURGICAL WOUNDS

0 International Council of Nurses (2011) defines a surgical wound as a "cut of tissue produced by a sharp surgical instrument in order to create an opening in a body space or organ, producing drainage of serum and blood, which is expected to be clean, i.e. without showing any signs of infection or pus". The surgical wound is the result of a planned procedure, whether in an elective or emergency context, and tissue healing is expected to follow a rapid, predictable evolution with minimal loss of function. People with surgical wounds should receive an appropriate assessment, as well as care appropriate to their clinical situation. This should begin in the preoperative period, continue in the intra- and postoperative periods and continue into outpatient care. Surgical wounds are classified according to the likelihood and degree of contamination of the wound at the time of the surgical intervention, following the definitions of the Centers for Disease Control and Prevention, of the World Health Organisation, and transposed into the DGS standard (2013).

3.2. CLASSIFICATION ACCORDING TO THE LIKELIHOOD AND DEGREE OF WOUND CONTAMINATION

Surgical wounds can be classified as: Clean; Clean-contaminated; Contaminated; Dirty or infected.

The clean surgical wound - This is the surgical wound resulting from elective, non-traumatic, non-infected surgery in which there has been no violation of surgical technique; there has been no penetration of the respiratory, digestive or genitourinary tract;

The clean-contaminated surgical wound - This is the surgical wound from operations in which the respiratory, digestive or genitourinary system has been penetrated under controlled conditions (correct surgical technique) and without contamination or evidence of infection;

Contaminated surgical wounds - These are surgical wounds from operations involving serious breaches of surgical technique; traumatic wounds; or those in which the respiratory, digestive or genitourinary system has been penetrated in the presence of infection;

A dirty or infected surgical wound - This is a traumatic wound with devitalised tissue, foreign bodies, faecal contamination, the presence of pus, perforated wounds or wounds where surgical treatment was delayed.

3.3. CLASSIFICATION ACCORDING TO THE HEALING PROCESS

In terms of the healing process, wounds can heal by first intention, second intention, third intention or biological coverings.

3.3.1. Healing by first intention

It refers to the approximation of wound edges by manual sutures, staples, clips or plastic skin.

This type of healing can be jeopardised by the presence of infection or foreign bodies.

The aim is to approximate each layer of skin, muscle and subcutaneous cell tissue in order to accelerate haemostasis and the healing mechanism (Yao et al., 2013).

The aim of this treatment is to restore physical integrity without infection and with minimal deformities.

Healing continues for the next 7 to 14 days and there are usually no complications.

According to NICE (2008), clean wounds should be closed immediately to allow healing by first intention.

After 48 hours, surgical wounds may only need cleaning and protection, which is easy to teach to the patient and their family.

3.3.2. Healing by second intention

It corresponds to wounds with extensive tissue loss and large surfaces. Wounds are opened and closed by the gradual process of granulation, contraction and epithelialisation.

In second intention healing, the surgical wound can either be left open intentionally at the time of surgery (so that it heals "naturally" by granulation, contraction and epithelialisation) or it can be opened after surgery.

Leaving wounds open is an option whenever closure is considered harmful. This type of healing can be used, for example, in abscesses, pilonidal sinuses or extensive wounds, such as abrasions, when closure by first intention is impossible (Moore and Foster, 2000).

It is important to emphasise that surgical wounds can be left open for a variety of reasons, including: considerable tissue loss (e.g. radical vulvectomy), a flat incision (shallow) but with a large surface area (e.g. donor sites), sites where there is infection (e.g. ruptured appendix) or an abscess that needs to be drained free of pus (Dealey, 2005).

There are cases in which surgical wounds open accidentally after they were originally closed (dehiscence occurs). In these cases, the wounds are usually left to heal by second intention and treatment should be carried out according to the type of wound involved. Due to the length of time and the healing process, these wounds can be considered chronic and their treatment is identical to this type of wound;

3.3.3. Healing by third intention

In third intention healing, the wound is left open for a certain period of time, with the intention of closing it surgically afterwards. In this way, the edges of the wound are brought back together at a later stage.

3.3.4. Healing by bio/6gic coverings

Healing takes place by applying free flaps of skin to the wound surface, or free or pedicled grafts of skin and subcutaneous cell tissue, which can be repositioned to facilitate healing.

3.4. PHASES OF THE HEALING PROCESS

These phases generally follow one another, but there can be overlapping phases in different locations of the wound, and the length of time each phase lasts can vary according to multiple factors.

3.4.1. Vascu/ar phase (in a few minutes)

In chronic wounds, the vascular phase may be absent. If the wound bleeds, to stop the bleeding the blood vessels contract due to the vascular smooth muscle itself (myogenic contraction) or due to the release of catecholamines from the sympathetic nervous system of these vessels (neurogenic contraction). This contraction lasts a maximum of one minute, which is enough time to stem the loss of blood fluid and start the coagulation process.

This process is accelerated by platelet aggregation and the release of various growth factors necessary for wound repair. Coagulation is preceded by a complex chain reaction called the coagulation cascade that leads to the formation of a clot, the main constituent of which i s fibrin, capable of trapping other blood cells. This gradual drying leads to the formation of the wound's crust, at the same time as the peripheral vasodilation begins to occur.

3.4.2. Infant/amateur phase (0-3 days)

In the case of chronic wounds, two phenomena occur during this phase: haemostasis and inflammation.

In acute wounds, only inflammation occurs.
Haemostasis:

• Trauma occurs;

• Vasoconstriction (damaged blood cells) = Haemostasis, if longer than 60 minutes, and if there is an associated pathology;
• Fibrin-reinforced platelet agglutinate = fibrin coagulum.

Inflammation:

• Release of histamine and other mediators = response of damaged tissue;

• Vasodilation of intact blood vessels;

• Increased blood flow = heat and flushing;

• Increased capillary permeability;

• Protein-rich fluid passes into the interstitial space;

• Local oedema = swelling and pain;

• Polymorphs, mast cells and macrophages are released at the site of the lesion as response to aggressive agents.
The inflammatory phase is vital for stimulating the following phases, hence the difficulty of healing in immunosuppressed patients.

In clean wounds, this phase can last around 36 hours; in necrotic or infected wounds, it can last longer.

3.4.3. Destructive phase (1-6 days)

In the destructive phase, the wound bed is cleaned of dead / devitalised tissue.

• 1° neutrophils (phagocytosis, 6 hours after trauma up to two to three days),

• 2° monocytes (arise due to the release of growth factors) and when they mature, they give way to macrophages (48 hours after the trauma), which are largely responsible for the healing process.

Polymorphs are responsible for phagocytosis and eliminate bacteria.

Macrophages stimulate the formation of fibroblasts, which in turn stimulate the production of collagen; they destroy bacteria and remove devitalised tissue and excess fibrin, producing factors that stimulate angiogenesis. The polymorphs and macrophages decrease their activity with a drop in thetemperature, their activity is inhibited by hypoxia and poor blood perfusion.

3.4.4. Pro/iferative phase (3-24 days)

Fibroblasts stimulate the production of collagen and an underlying substance. This substance causes an underlying inflammation.

Angiogenesis promotes the elimination of fibrin clots and the formation of neovascularisation (capillaries) due to the presence of specific enzymes.

The resulting collagen and neovascularisation produce circumvallations of capillaries (very fragile and easily damaged), supported by the underlying substance, resulting in granulation tissue. This phase becomes slower with age. Vitamin C is essential for collagen synthesis.

3.4.5. Maturation stage (24-365 days)

The wound is filled with new connective tissue by the following processes:

• Granulation;

• Contraction;

• Epithelialisation.
At the same time as granulation tissue is formed, connective tissue is produced (contraction and epithelialisation). Collagen fibres thicken and reorganise themselves. Tensile strength increases. The wound bed becomes pale and less vascularised. The epithelial cells migrate over the granulation tissue.

Cell division ceases when the cells meet due to contact inhibition, the wound contracts due to the contractile capacity of the microblasts, the wound edges join together.

But pay attention:

• Wound contraction is useful, but can be unsightly, for example on the neck and face;

• If the edges of the wound are damaged, the wound may contract.

inhibited;

• The resulting skin is very vulnerable;

• Epithelialisation is three times faster in a humid environment.

3.5. FACTORS INFLUENCING HEALING

• **Blood supply** - Alterations in peripheral blood supply reduce tissue perfusion, compromising local oxygenation and nutrient supply.

• **Oxygenation** - Hypoxia stimulates angiogenesis, but adequate oxygenation is needed at the wound margins. Low oxygen levels stimulate collagen synthesis, epithelial growth and decrease the tissue's resistance to infection due to loss of neutrophil phagocytic capacity. Oxygen levels in the wound can be measured by transcutaneous assessment.

• **Nutrition** - Essential for the functioning of the immune system, preventing infection and promoting healing. Protein, calories, vitamin A and E, zinc, arginine and glutamine are some of the important elements.

• **Temperature fluctuations** - Mitotic activity occurs more rapidly at body temperature. Extreme temperatures cause tissue damage).

• **Associated pathologies** - such as diabetes, immunological diseases, vascular insufficiencies.

• **Associated medication** - Corticoids have an anti-inflammatory, anti-mitotic effect, decrease the synthesis of matrix components and delay epithelialisation. Vitamin A may counteract this effect by mechanisms that have not yet been clarified.

• **Dehydration** - Epithelialisation, contraction and granulation of the wound occur more quickly in a humid environment than in a dry one.

• **Wound location** - Affects healing, closed wounds heal more slowly.

• **Age of the wound** - Chronic wounds are by definition difficult to heal, prolonged healing times require investigation.

• **Foreign bodies** - cause tissue irritation, prolong inflammation and can increase infection - gas leftovers, sutures, bone fragments and necrotic tissue.

• **Necrotic tissue** - prevents epithelial and nutrient migration to the wound bed.

• **Skin maceration** - Excessive exudate, sweating or incontinence can cause infection, sensitisation and skin irritation.

• **Surgical technique** - Excessive scar tissue, inadequate wound drainage.

4. PERILESIONAL SKIN CARE

The skin's main function is to protect against the entry of microorganisms, water and trauma. Preventing damage to the skin is one of the primary objectives of healthcare professionals in the prevention and treatment of wounds.

Preserving the integrity of the skin requires an appropriate approach based on four fundamental areas:

• Cleaning,

• Moisturising,

• Protection

• Continuity of care.

To maintain clean skin, we recommend using water and soap with a neutral pH to wash with a soft cloth or sponge and towel to dry.

As the body's defence mechanisms are sometimes unable to manage the factors that put the skin at risk, particularly humidity, the products normally used to maintain this balance fall into two families: barrier creams and emollients.

Despite the fact that these products have different functions, there are still professional

who do not use them properly.

Emollients form an inert barrier under the skin's surface, trapping moisture underneath. These products help to reduce water loss through the skin. They come in various forms: lotions, creams, oils, bath additives and soap substitutes (Hampton, 2004). Barrier creams are products used to protect the skin against aggressions caused by excessive exposure to water, exudate or irritants (e.g. faeces, urine, sweating, drainage...).

The basic composition of a barrier cream consists of a lipophilic/water emulsion with an addition of metallic or titanic oxide (Voegeli, 2008).

There are now new generation products that allow a thin layer of semi-permeable protective polymer to be applied. According to Voegeli (2008), this type of product represents added value in promoting the protection of perilesional skin and, consequently, an improvement in the quality of care, reflected in the greater satisfaction of users and the professionals who provide this healthcare.

The effectiveness of wound care depends on the ability to manage the exudate produced by the wound, seeking to achieve a balance of moisture at the wound-primary dressing interface, exudate released in the form of water vapour, and that retained in the medical device, thus reducing the risk of dehydration and maceration.

Prolonged contact with moisture also inhibits the skin's barrier function, increasing the risk of maceration, skin breakdown, exogenous eczema and contact dermatitis.

The production of wound exudate is the result of vasodilation during the inflammatory phase, influenced by mediators such as histamine and bradykinin. It is part of the healing process and appears as serous content in the wound bed. In chronic wounds, the inflammation is persistent and long-lasting, and an infectious process may or may not set in, leading to changes in the exudate that generate some clinical challenges.

In chronic wounds, high exudate degrades growth factors by increasing the concentration of metalloproteinases (MMPs), delaying the healing process and making it difficult to select a treatment (Gonzalez, F.; Fornells, M. 2009).

5. IMPORTANCE OF WOUND EXUDATE

The exudate from a wound is important because:

• Maintains moisture in the wound;

• Helps repair cells migrate;

• It transports nutrients, among other things.

There is no one treatment for controlling wound exudate, but its selection must always take into account the acronym TIME, i.e. the type of tissue in the wound, the existence of inflammation or infection, the quantity and type of exudate and the edges of the wound (Gonzalez, F.; Fornells, M. 2009).

The acronym "TIME" is the result of dividing the wound bed preparation process into its components in a reproducible way:

• "T" refers to the removal of non-viable tissue;

• "I" refers to infection control and the reduction of the bacterial load;

• "M" is the maintenance of moisture balance, as the wound must be kept moist, but not excessively exudative;

• "E" refers to the migration of keratin6cites in the wound bed.

The characteristics of the exudate produced by the wound condition the selection of the medical device to be used.

When treating wounds, in patients with fragile, oedematous or macerated skin, dressings with vertical absorption capacity should be applied, with unconventional adhesive edges (silicone) and perilesional protection should always be provided with a barrier cream.

It should always be borne in mind that the effectiveness of a dressing can be affected by the effect of friction and sliding forces, depending on the region where the wound is located, and can lead to an additional wound due to the leakage of exudate or maceration of the perilesional skin, which can be extremely painful and slow down the healing process, requiring immediate treatment. It is essential to adopt clinical practices based on scientific evidence, with therapeutic approaches and using medical devices appropriate to the situations identified.

6. NUTRITION IN WOUND CARE

Nutrition plays an essential role in the prevention, treatment and healing of wounds. Nutritional care is an integral part of all health care. When nutritional status is compromised, before or during the healing process, the entire physiological healing process (all phases) is compromised: it is longer or impossible, more painful and costly and, if not complete, more likely to recur and become chronic. Chronic wounds particularly affect the elderly, diabetics and/or people with other chronic diseases, and represent a huge burden on society and the health system.In situations of insufficient food supply, particularly protein, and in the presence of wounds or disease, "muscle tissue autophagy" can occur in order to obtain the proteins (amino acids) needed for protein synthesis, which occurs in the healing process of a wound. This metabolic process also requires the presence of other nutrients, micronutrients (vitamins and minerals) and energy.If the energy supply from food is not sufficient, muscle tissue proteins (lean mass) are also catabolised into glucose (energy), further aggravating the state of malnutrition. However, when the loss of lean mass is severe, and death is imminent, the "host" favours survival over injury. With a loss of 20 per cent or more of lean mass, the wound "competes" with the muscle to recruit nutrients from the diet for healing. If the loss of lean mass is greater than 30%, the reconstruction of muscle is prioritised over healing.Body composition can change before a wound and it certainly changes after a wound. Nutrition is a determining factor in the health care process. Therefore, assessing nutritional status is mandatory before, in the case of planned surgical wounds, during, or after the appearance of the wound. The objectives of nutritional care are defined according to the person, not the wound. There are no nutritional recommendations for wounds, but rather nutritional recommendations for different people with different wounds.

The aim of nutritional care is to

• Providing an adequate energy supply, with a view to maximising nitrogen retention;

• Provide the necessary protein intake to promote a positive nitrogen balance;

• Avoiding the loss of lean mass and preventing its replacement by adipose tissue;

• Provide at least 100 per cent of nutritional needs for micronutrients (vitamins and minerals) every day;

• Monitor the nutritional outcomes of the food provided, particularly biochemicals, to avoid toxicity associated with excessive intake;

• Suspecting, confirming and treating nutritional deficiencies, particularly of

vitamins A and C and Zn;

• Achieving and maintaining optimal hydration and perfusion of wounded tissues;

• Achieving and maintaining glycaemic control;

• Monitor proposed food intake;

• Adjust the current nutritional intervention to the desired nutritional intervention;

• Adjust the nutritional care plan with a view to the desired and expected end results.

The response to nutritional care depends on the etiology, severity, location, extent, number of wounds and the clinical situation prior to the appearance of the wound, the current clinical situation, as well as the patient's previous or current nutritional status.

Non-nutritional factors that affect the healing process:

• advanced age;

• Ambient temperature above 30°C;

• Anti-inflammatory medication;

• Chemotherapy and radiotherapy;

• Concomitant chronic diseases, such as diabetes, liver, kidney, vascular or autoimmune disease;

• Inflammatory disease;

• Type of material used in the dressing;

• Presence of foreign bodies in the wound;

• Hyp6xia at the wound site;

• Concomitant presence of local or systemic infection;

• Urinary and faecal incontinence;

• Mobility;

• Presence of necrotic tissue;

• Nonspecific metabolic changes;

• Cancer, sepsis or other catabolic situations;

• Specific surgical techniques.

Energy and nutritional needs depend on the individual, their age, the stage of the life cycle they are in, their physical activity, their weight, their intention to lose or gain weight.

But nutritional needs also depend on the individual's nutritional status, the disease and the wound. According to the EPUAP (European Pressure Ulcer Advisory Panel) and NPUAP (National Pressure Ulcer Advisory Panel) recommendations for pressure ulcers, published in 2009, energy requirements should be determined on the basis of 30-35 Kcal/Kg current weight/day. They should be adjusted for cases in which weight loss has previously occurred, or in the presence of overweight/obesity.

7. ASSESSMENT AND CHARACTERISATION OF WOUNDS

The diagnostic process of a person with a wound must be considered the starting point for effective and efficient treatment. The assessment and characterisation of wounds is one of the elements of diagnosis, which must be multidimensional and integrate knowledge of skin anatomy and physiology, healing physiology and wound etiopathogenesis.

Being multidimensional, the diagnosis must be based on:

• Anamnesis;

• Physical examination;

• Evaluation / characterisation of the wound and peri-lesional skin.
Bearing in mind the multidimensionality of all the diagnostic elements, we have to take them into account:

• Pain assessment;

• Nutritional assessment;

• Quality of life assessment;

• Assessment of conditions / risk factors;

• Psychosocial assessment.
Aspects to consider when assessing wounds:

• **Etiology** - Surgical wounds are intentional and can heal by first intention, second intention or delayed first intention. Traumatic wounds are usually accidental: abrasions, cuts, punctures, crushing, animal bites and burns. Difficult-to-heal wounds are pressure ulcers, diabetic feet, leg ulcers, cancer wounds and atypical wounds. Difficult-to-heal wounds have an inherent irreversibility that is influenced multifactorially by

"

personal (physical and psychosocial), biochemical and microbiological variables,

The causal, etiological factor, "repeated trauma", also plays a major role in its development.

• **Localisation** - The localisation of a wound can be an indicator of its etiology. There are wounds that often develop in certain anatomical locations. However, this should not be considered the sole defining characteristic of the aetiology. The location of the wound should be based on anatomical models and described in precise, classified language.

• **Dimensions** - The characterisation of a wound according to its dimensions should include: length, width and depth. The size, depth and duration of the wound are three predictors of its evolution. There are several types of wound measurement: simple measurement (length and width); wound delineator; planimetry; three-dimensional measurement (determines the volume of the wound); and photography.

• **Existence of locae, f1stulas and/or fistulous tracts** - These are conditions that make it difficult to assess the wound and, consequently, its treatment. This is why the assessment of dimensions requires a detailed exploration of the wound, albeit non-traumatic, in order to correctly diagnose and characterise the existence of any of these alterations. Their existence is usually identified using the idea of a clock to make an analogy of the wound, thus defining the location of the site and/or path and also determining its depth, if possible.

• **Exudate** - Exudate must be characterised in terms of colour, quantity and consistency. In terms of colour, it can be: serous (yellow); bloody (red); or serous-bloody (yellowish with traces of blood). With regard to quantity, it can be: little, moderate or abundant. In terms of consistency, it can be: fluid, thick or purulent.

• **Odour** - Odour can be classified as present or absent. The presence of odour can be indicative of colonisation or infection.

• **Pain** - It is important to identify and classify pain. Understanding whether it exists, how, when and with what intensity is fundamental in the assessment process and in the wound healing/treatment process. Pain is a frequent symptom in patients with a wide variety of wounds. In order to carry out this assessment, it is important to know the physiology of pain and its classification. Pain can be: nociceptive, neuropathic or idiopathic. It can also be classified as acute or chronic. When assessing and treating a person with a wound, it is essential to understand that pain is more than nociception, more than a sensation; it is an unpleasant, individual, personal and subjective experience. According to the European Wound Management Association (EWMA, 2002), studies related to quality of life have consistently shown that pain improves significantly with effective treatments that promote healing. To assess and characterise pain in the area of wound care, there are a wide variety of scales: visual analogue scale, numerical scale, qualitative verbal scale and face scale. Best practice in local treatment, drug therapy and other complementary approaches should be taken into account when dealing with and controlling pain.

• **Tissue type/wound bed** - The wound bed and the type of tissue present are indicative of the stage of healing, its progression and the effectiveness of the treatment. Depending on the type of tissue present, the objectives and local therapeutic measures are also different. In addition to the type of tissue, when assessing the wound bed we must also consider aspects such as exudate, size (for example, whether it is cavitating or not), whether it shows signs of infection, which can lead to different types of tissue and conditions coexisting. The wound bed can have different types of tissue:

o **Necrosis**: usually black in colour, indicative of devitalisation and can have a hard or soft consistency;

o **Fibrin**: yellowish in colour and may adhere to the wound bed;

o **Granulation**: reddish-coloured tissue which, at the same time, if slightly moist and firm, is indicative of good progress in the healing process;

o **Epithelialisation**: pinkish tissue, indicative of wound closure and which therefore usually emerges from the edges of the wound.

• **Wound edges and peri-lesional skin** - The condition of the wound edges and peri-lesional skin is important for wound closure. Healthy surrounding skin favours epithelialisation and wound closure.

Changes such as maceration, erythema, oedema, eczema or cellulitis are detrimental to the healing process. Their diagnosis and treatment are crucial as they can be indicative of alterations in the healing process (e.g. infection), inadequate local treatment or non-existent additional care (e.g. pressure relief).

• **Signs of critical colonisation/infection** - Wounds are naturally colonised, but states of critical colonisation and infection delay, stagnate or prevent the healing process and can have serious systemic consequences if left unchecked. Wound assessment is a multidimensional process that must be systematised and systematic. Reassessment should be carried out frequently and if changes in appetite are detected, the therapeutic plan should be reassessed and altered if necessary. Records should be kept in accordance with the information systems in force. Photographic recording, with informed consent, is a useful complement in parameterising and assessing the wound.

8.   PRODUCTS WITH THERAPEUTIC ACTION

In order to select the best therapeutic option, knowledge of the available products must be as complete as possible, combined with comprehensive knowledge of the physiology of healing and a holistic approach to the person with the wound.

• **Hyperoxygenated fatty acids** - Composed of essential fatty acids, mainly linoleic acid. They increase skin hydration by replenishing the hydrolipidic film and blood microcirculation through capillary renewal, favouring skin elasticity and resistance. They are indicated for the prevention of pressure ulcers and the treatment of category I pressure ulcers. They come in spray and capsule form. They are applied to the whole skin and gently massaged in until the product is completely absorbed, repeating the procedure two or three times a day.

• **Hyaluronic acid** - Hyaluronic acid is a natural polysaccharide molecule found in the extracellular matrix of various tissues and organs in the body. It plays an important role in all phases of the healing process, especially in chronic wounds that are not progressing. It has an effect on the organisation of proteoglycans, on the proliferation of granulation tissue by facilitating angiogenesis and the formation of connective tissue and on cell migration, particularly of keratin6cites. In contact with the wound, it turns into a hydrophilic gel, promoting a moist environment that favours healing. It is contraindicated in critically colonised and infected wounds. It comes in the form of sheets, ampoules, strips and microgranules. It can remain on the wound for up to three days.

• **Alginates** - Alginates are natural polysaccharides derived from alginic acid extracted from seaweed. They act by ion exchange between the calcium ions in the alginate and the sodium ions in the wound exudate. In contact with this, they form a gel which creates a moist environment that favours healing, promotes autolytic debridement and relieves pain (by moistening the nerve endings). They also have a haemostatic effect by inducing the formation of prothrombin through calcium ions. They are useful on infected wounds as they which have a bacteriostatic effect by retaining microorganisms in their structure. They are indicated for extremely exuding wounds, both superficial and deep, as they have an absorption capacity of ten to twenty times their weight. However, they absorb exudate longitudinally, which is why it is recommended that their application should not extend beyond the edges of the wound. They are not useful in the presence of dry necrosis or poorly exuding wounds. It is the amount of exudate that indicates how long they should remain on the wound, which can be up to seven days. They require secondary application. They come in the form of sheets and strips; the strips are suitable for cavitary and deep wounds.

• **Activated charcoal ap6sites** - Charcoal has a deodorising effect because it adsorbs the molecules responsible for bad odours to the surface. When combined with silver, it is indicated for infected wounds due to the antimicrobial effect of silver. In association with alginates and carboxymethylcellulose, they are useful for exuding wounds due to their absorption power. Some applications cannot be cut due to the risk of releasing charcoal particles. They can remain in the wound for up to seven days depending on the properties of the secondary ap6site.

• **Collagenase** - Collagenase is an exogenous enzyme with recognised functions in the enzymatic debridement of necrotic tissue. It works by destroying fibrin, collagen and elastin, separating necrotic tissue from viable tissue. It comes in the form of an ointment. It requires secondary application and can be combined with a hydrogel. It can cause a sensitivity reaction in the perilesional skin, which is why it must be protected beforehand. Contraindicated on infected wounds. Soaps, detergents, antiseptics and heavy metals should not be used as they inactivate collagenase. Dressings should be changed daily and may remain on the wound for longer if combined with a hydrogel, depending on the condition of the perilesional skin and the associated secondary wound.

• **Collagen ap6sites** - Collagen is a protein found in the skin that plays an important role in the healing process, as it stimulates the growth of granulation tissue by stimulating angiogenesis and the development of fibroblasts. It also has a haemostatic action by increasing aggregation platelets. It is indicated for chronic, unevolved wounds, ideally without necrosis and/or infection. It should be used with secondary ap6sites (e.g. foams). It comes in the form of powder, granules or plaques. May be associated with other substances such as protease modelling matrix and gentamicin. It does not need to be removed because it is absorbed.

• **Acrylic copolymer** - A polymeric solution that forms a uniform film when applied to the skin, with the ability to prevent and treat the effects of excess moisture caused by incontinence, digestive juices and wound exudates, as well as adhesives and rubbing products. It comes in the form of a spray that doesn't transfer to other surfaces, such as nappies and dressing material, allowing for increased adhesion of products. For the protection of perilesional skin, the frequency of application varies depending on the amount and type of exudate and can last from 48 to 72 hours.

• **Polyurethane foams** - Composed of hydrocellular foams with hydrophilic substances. They have a high capacity to absorb exudate (even under compression), reducing the risk of maceration of the perilesional skin as they do not gel when in contact with exudate. They are absorbed horizontally. They are indicated as primary dressings in wounds undergoing granulation and epithelialisation, and as secondary dressings associated with other dressing materials such as hydrogels in wounds with necrosis. Some can be used to reduce pressure and prevent pressure ulcers. They come with and without an adhesive border, in various specific anatomical shapes (e.g. sacrococcygeal area and calcaneus) and in the form of spherical structures for cavitary wounds. They can remain in the wound for up to seven days and their frequency of change depends on the amount of exudate. They are also useful for hypergranulating wounds.

• **Polyurethane films** - Formed by a transparent, semi-permeable polyurethane sheet - permeable for gas exchange and impermeable to water and microorganisms. They have no absorption capacity. They are indicated as primary dressings on wounds without exudate and in the epithelialisation phase or for prevention on skin subject to friction. They are indicated as secondary dressings for fixing other dressing materials, such as, hydrogels. They are contraindicated on infected wounds. They can be left on for up to seven days.

• **Hydrocol6ides** - These are products made up of s6dical carboxymethylcellulose (CMC), proteins, gelatine and an outer polyurethane coating. When in contact with wound exudate, a gel is formed, with a characteristic (and somewhat unpleasant) colour and odour, which promotes autophthalmic debridement. They have a low to moderate capacity for absorbing exudate. Because they are occlusive, they constitute a mechanical barrier to bacterial contamination, but are contraindicated in infected wounds. They are indicated for wounds with little exudate, in granulation, epithelialisation and as a secondary dressing. It is also indicated as a preventative method in areas subject to friction. They come in the form of a plaque, with various dimensions and specific anatomical shapes (e.g. sacrococcygeal region) with or without a border. The frequency of dressing changes is determined by the amount of exudate, with a maximum stay of seven days.

• **Hydrofibres** - Composed of sodium carboxymethylcellulose. They have a high absorption capacity and can absorb up to thirty times their own weight. Absorption takes place vertically and the exudate is retained, transforming it into a gel and preventing maceration of the perilesional tissue. They are indicated for moderate to extremely exuding wounds. They are useful in wounds with fistulous tracts and in cavities where the filling should not exceed 80% of the wound area. They promote a moist environment which, in addition to reducing pain, enhances autolytic debridement. They require secondary application. They can remain on the wound for up to seven days or be changed earlier if saturated.

• **Hydrogels** - Composed essentially of water (70% to 90%) and other crystalline systems of polysaccharides and synthetic polymers. They promote tissue rehydration, favouring autophthalmic debridement and contributing to angiogenesis, granulation and epithelialisation. Their use in combination with collagenase enhances the debridement effect. Due to its moisturising action, it helps to reduce pain locally by moisturising the nerve endings and because it doesn't adhere to the wound bed, it allows it to be removed from the wound.

Atraumatic removal. Particularly recommended for wounds with necrosis, it can also be used on granulation and epithelialisation tissues. On necrotic plaques, it is necessary to make some cuts with a scalpel in criss-cross lines to allow the product to penetrate and consequently moisturise the tissues. There are various presentations: amorphous gel, mesh and plaque. In gel and/or mesh form, it is necessary to use a secondary dressing (hydrocol6ide or hydropolymer, depending on the amount of exudate). Dressings can be changed every three days or according to the condition of the wound.

• **Ap6sites with iodine** - Iodine has a broad antimicrobial spectrum and is effective in treating infections caused by Gram + and Gram - bacteria, fungi, viruses, spores and protozoa. It comes in the form of tulle impregnated with 10% povidone-iodine and gauze impregnated with iodine cadex6mer. The iodine is released in a controlled manner, and iodine cadex6mer is recommended for exuding wounds due to its greater absorption capacity – 1 g of iodine cadex6mer can absorb up to 6 ml of fluid, whereas tulle impregnated with povidone-iodine has no absorption capacity. Iodine cadex6mer also has debridement capabilities. Iodine is contraindicated in people with known sensitivity to iodine, Hashimoto's thyroiditis, multinodular goitre, children, and pregnant and breastfeeding women. They require secondary treatment. They can remain in the wound for three to four days depending on the amount of exudate.

• **Maltodextrin** - A natural product obtained by hydrolysis of carbohydrates. In contact with the wound bed, it enhances autophthalmic debridement, promotes a moist environment and provides the wound bed with nutrients necessary for the healing process. It comes in p6 or gel form, for application to wounds with exudate or dry necrosis, respectively. It can be applied to infected wounds and has the effect of reducing odour, as the decrease in pH provided by ascorbic acid limits the growth of microorganisms. Requires secondary dressing. Requires daily dressing. Can be used for up to 30 days after opening the packaging.

• **Ap6sites with honey** - Sterile ap6sites consisting mainly of honey. Recommended for critically colonised or infected wounds. Through the action of glucose oxidase, it causes the release of hydrogen peroxide in non-toxic doses with an antimicrobial effect. It controls acidity in the wound bed, maintaining a pH between three and five, which restricts the growth of various species of microorganisms. It has a broad spectrum and is effective in the presence of fungi, protozoa, Gram + and Gram – bacteria and those resistant to antibiotics (methylcillin-resistant

Staphylococcus aureus and multi-resistant Pseudomonas aeruginosa). The high osmolarity of honey can cause slight, passing pain after the honey is placed on the wound bed. Has an effect on odour control. Requires secondary application. Depending on the condition of the wound bed and the type of dressing, they can remain for up to three days.

• **Polyacrylate dressing** - Polyacrylate dressing with or without hyperosmolar Ringer's solution. In addition to the high absorption capacity conferred by polyacrylate, it promotes debridement through the action of Ringer's solution. It is indicated for debridement of dry necrotic tissues. It should not be applied beyond the edges of the wound due to the risk of maceration of the perilesional skin. It requires a secondary dressing, should not be cut and requires daily dressing changes. Polyacrylate dressings, but without ringer's solution, can be used as a primary dressing, or before the secondary dressing, in order to increase absorption capacity. They are indicated for moderate to very exuding wounds. They cannot be cut.

• **Ap6site with polyhexanide** - Polyhexanide has a broad antimicrobial spectrum that is effective against aer6bial and anaer6bial bacteria, MRSA and VRE, fungi and yeasts. It is indicated for the treatment of critically colonised and infected wounds. It comes in the form of an irrigation solution, gel, sheets and strips. The sheets and strips consist of cellulose fibres associated with polyhexamethylene biguanide (PHMB) and can remain on the wound for up to seven days. In addition to its antimicrobial effect, the gel has a debridement effect. It can be used for eight weeks after opening. They require secondary application.

• **Ap6site with silver** - Ap6sites impregnated with silver in different percentages and associated with different materials (hydrocol6ides, polyurethane, activated charcoal, hydrofibres and alginates) suited to the conditions of the wound bed and the amount of exudate. Silver has a bactericidal action, as it acts by causing structural changes in the bacterial cell wall and membranes without damaging human cells. It is effective in infections caused by a wide range of microorganisms, including multi-resistant ones such as Pseudomonas aeruginosa, Staphylococcus aureus and Candida albicans. It has no known side effects and produces little resistance. For these reasons, it is indicated for critically colonised and/or infected wounds. Most dressings release silver in its ionic form into the wound bed in a controlled and gradual manner, with the exception of silver-activated charcoal dressings, which adsorb exudate and inactivate bacteria in contact with the dressing.

• **Silicone dressings** - These are mostly composed of silicone. Their main characteristic is that they do not adhere to the wound bed, allowing them to be removed without traumatising the newly formed tissue or causing pain. They are indicated for wounds in the granulation phase, wounds where there is a lot of adherence of other substances and wounds where the perilesional tissue is weakened, as they are fluid repellent and do not adhere to the wound, but to the surrounding area without damaging it. They come in the form of tulle, sheets and in combination with polyurethane foams. Plaques are useful for preventing colloids and improving the aesthetic results of healing. When combined with foams, it provides vertical absorption.

• **Ap6sites impregnated with petrolatum, paraffin or lanolin** - Ap6sites impregnated with petrolatum, paraffin or lanolin, especially suitable for wounds that are not very exuding and are in the granulation or epithelialisation phase. One of their main effects is to protect newly formed tissue, especially from adhering ap6sites, and to minimise pain when changing the dressing. They can remain on the wound for one to three days.

9. WOUND CLEANING AND/OR DISINFECTION PROCEDURE

In order to select the best therapeutic option, knowledge of the available products must be as complete as possible, combined with comprehensive knowledge of the physiology of healing and a holistic approach to the person with the wound.

"The wound dressing procedure consists of cleaning or disinfecting the skin and underlying tissues and, if necessary, applying a protective dressing" with the aims of: Promoting wound healing; Protecting the skin and underlying tissues; Preventing infection; Draining the contents of the wound and Maintaining comfort and well-being (ACSS, 2011; page 64).

Before carrying out the procedure, it is important to follow some guidelines such as:

• Consult the clinical file to individualise, diagnose, plan care and evaluate results;
• Check the environmental conditions: temperature, ventilation and lighting;

• Respect the client's privacy;

• Observe the client: face, posture, smell of the wound, among other signs;

• Examining the client: pain, well-being;

• Provide advice on hygiene and site protection;

• Arrange for the wound to be treated in an appropriate place whenever possible;
• Prepare the material according to the type of wound and the client's needs (e.g. surgical wound, trauma wound, ulcers, etc.);
• Perform with aseptic technique and using a mask, if indicated;

• Clean the wound, from the least contaminated area to the most contaminated;

• Wash chronic wounds and the surrounding area in order to remove all dirt;

• Avoid friction when cleaning the wound, using minimal mechanical force to prevent trauma to the healing tissues;

• Treat the wound with gentle movements in order to prevent

accidental failure of drains or drainage systems;

• Use circular movements to clean the drain from the proximal to the distal area;

• Treat the wound whenever the dressing is wet,

overwritten, detached or soiled, to prevent the proliferation of micro-organisms;

• Apply isotonic sodium chloride at a temperature of no less than 28°C;

• Apply the dressing leaving a 3cm margin of intact skin.

As materials, we can use a dressing tray or trolley with a dressing kit, sterile and non-sterile gloves, isotonic sodium chloride, sterile dressing, adhesive, non-sterile scissors, disposable gauze, a dirty container. If necessary, we can use an antiseptic, sterile scissors, sterile bowl, forceps for removing staples, dissecting forceps, Kocher forceps, sterile compresses, ligature/tube net, sterile pin, drain or drainage system and catheter of suitable calibre, syringe and mask.

9.1. PROCEDURE FOR SURGICAL WOUNDS

According to the ACSS guidelines (2011), nursing actions for surgical wounds include

1) Provide resources to the client to manage time;

2) Wash your hands to prevent infection;

3) Educate the client about the procedure in order to get their co-operation and reduce anxiety;
4) Position the client or assist them to position themselves, according to their clinical situation and the area to be exposed, to facilitate the procedure;
5) Apply the waterproof covering under the customer;

6) Put on non-sterile gloves;

7) Remove the dressing;

8) Observe the characteristics of theremoved dressing, the wound and the surrounding area to monitor healing progress;
9) Remove gloves;

10) Wash your hands to prevent contamination; 11)Prepare the dressing kit and/or sterilised material;
12) Put on sterilised gloves if necessary;

13) Clean or irrigate the wound to remove micro-organisms, prevent infection and tissue damage and favour healing;
14) Remove dots/staples if indicated;

15) Mobilise, fix or remove the drain, if necessary; 16)Observe the characteristics of the drained contents;
17) Clean the wound;

18) Clean the area around the wound with sterile compresses and apply a dressing to prevent contamination and facilitate adherence of the dressing;
19) Position or assist the client to position themselves to avoid putting pressure on an area whose skin integrity is altered;

20) Remove gloves if necessary;

21) Appreciate the client's well-being and facilitate the updating of the nursing diagnosis;

22) Collecting and washing material

23) Wash hands to prevent cross-transmission of microorganisms

24) Record: the date and time of the procedure, the nursing diagnoses, the nursing interventions, the results obtained and the health education carried out.

9.2. PROCEDURE FOR TRAUMATIC WOUNDS

According to the ACSS guidelines (2011), the nursing actions for wounds are traumatic:

1) Provide resources to the client to manage time;

2) Wash your hands to prevent infection;

3) Educate the client about the procedure in order to get their co-operation and reduce anxiety;

4) Position the client or assist them to position themselves, according to their clinical situation and the area to be exposed, to facilitate the procedure;

5) Apply the waterproof covering under the customer;

6) Put on non-sterile gloves;

7) Remove the dressing;

8) Observe the characteristics of theremoved dressing, the wound and the surrounding area to monitor healing progress;

9) Remove gloves;

10) Wash your hands to prevent contamination; 11)Prepare the dressing

kit and/or sterilised material;

12) Put on sterilised gloves if necessary;

13) Collect exudate for analysis, if necessary, in order t o   identify the presence of microorganisms;

14) Clean the wound or irrigate to remove microorganisms, prevent infection and favour healing;

15) Observe wound characteristics and monitor healing progress;

16) Clean the area around the wound with a sterilised compress to prevent contamination and facilitate adherence of the dressing;

17) Remove devitalised tissue, if necessary, to promote healing;

18) Re-irrigate the lesion and surrounding area with isotonic sodium chloride to remove residual devitalised tissue;

19) Ensure that the surrounding skin is dry, using a sterile compress to prevent contamination and facilitate adherence of the dressing;

20) Apply medication, if prescribed, to promote wound healing;

21) Protect the surrounding skin if necessary, avoiding maceration of the skin;

22) Apply a dressing, favouring contact with the topical agent, absorbing excess exudate and protecting the lesion from contamination;

23) Position or assist the client to position themselves, avoiding pressure on an area whose skin integrity is altered;

24) Remove gloves if necessary;

25) Appreciate the client's well-being and facilitate the updating of the nursing diagnosis;

26) Ensure that the material is collected and washed;

27) Wash hands to prevent cross-transmission of microorganisms;

28) Record: the date and time of the procedure, the nursing diagnoses,

the nursing interventions, the results obtained and the health education carried out.

9.3. PROCEDURE FOR ULCER WOUNDS

According to the ACSS guidelines (2011), the nursing actions for wounds are are traumatic:

1) Provide resources to the client to manage time;

2) Wash your hands to prevent infection;

3) Educate the client about the procedure in order to get their co-operation and reduce anxiety;

4) Position the client or assist them to position themselves, according to their clinical situation and the area to be exposed, to facilitate the procedure;

5) Apply the waterproof covering under the customer;

6) Put on non-sterile gloves;

7) Remove the dressing;

8) Observe the characteristics of theremoved dressing, the wound and the surrounding area to monitor healing progress;

9) Remove gloves;

10) Wash your hands to prevent contamination; 11)Prepare the dressing kit and/or sterile material;

12) Put on sterilised gloves if necessary;

13) Collect exudate for analysis and, if necessary, identify the presence of microorganisms;

14) Clean the wound to remove micro-organisms, prevent infection and promote healing;

15) Monitor the characteristics of the wound to assess signs of

progression;

16) Remove devitalised tissue, if indicated;

17) Irrigate the lesion and surrounding area with isotonic sodium chloride
to remove residual necrotic tissue;
18) Dry the lesion and surrounding skin with a sterile compress to prevent
contamination and facilitate adherence of the dressing;
19) Apply typical substances, if prescribed, to facilitate the removal of
necrotic tissue and healing;
20) Protect surrounding skin if necessary;

21) Apply a suitable dressing to facilitate contact with the toxic substance,
absorb excess exudate and protect the lesion from contamination;

22) Position or assist the client to position themselves, avoiding pressure
on an area whose skin integrity has been altered;
23) Remove gloves if necessary;

24) Appreciate the client's well-being and facilitate the updating of the
nursing diagnosis;
25) Ensure that the material is collected and washed;

26) Wash hands to prevent cross-transmission of microorganisms;

27) Record: the date and time of the procedure, the nursing diagnoses,
the nursing interventions, the results obtained and the health education
carried out.

BIBLIOGRAPHY

Central Administration of the Health System. ACCS (2011). Nursing Standards Manual - Technical Procedures. Lisbon: Ministry of Health

Afonso, C., Afonso, G., Azevedo, M., Miranda, M., & Alves, P. (2014). Prevençao e Tratamento de Feridas Da Evidência à Pratica. (I. pinto, Eugénio e vieira, Ed.) (Hartmann). Portugal. ISBN 978-989-20-5133-8.

Aldini, N. N., Fini, M., & Giardino, R. (2008). From Hippocrates to Tissue Engineering: Surgical Strategies in Wound Treatment. World Journal of Surgery, 2114-2121.

Alves, P.; Vieira, M. (2009). Wound education: undergraduate training in health courses. Master's dissertation in Educational Planning and Management. Universidade Portucalense.

Alves, P.; Teixeira, A.; Albuquerque, L.; Borges, C.; Magalhaes, B.; Mendes, D.; Ramos, P. (2021). The Role of Nutrition in Wound Prevention and Treatment. Portuguese Wound Care Association. ISBN 978-989-53418-2-5

Cohen, M., Giladi, M., Mayo, A., & Shafir, R. (1998). The granulometer-- a pocket scale for the assessment of wound healing. Annals of plastic surgery, 40(6), 641-645. https://doi.org/10.1097/00000637-199806000-00012

Dealey, C. (2005). German Wound Surgeons 1450-1750. EWMA Journal, 48-51.
DGS (2013). Chronic wound infection prevention. Guideline no. 019/2013 of 23/12/2013. Accessed at: https://www.dgs.pt/directrizes-da-dgs/orientacoes-e- circulars-informative/orientação-n-0192013-de-23122013.aspx

European Wound Management Association (EWMA). Position
Document: Pain at wound dressing changes. London: MEP Ltd, 2002.

European Pressure Ulcer Advisory Panel and National Pressure Ulcer
Advisory Panel Prevention and Treatment of Pressure Ulcers: Quick
Reference Guide. [Serial online]. 2009 [Cited 26 October 2013].
Available at: URL: http://www.epuap.org/guidelines/.

FORNELLS, M.; GONZALEZ, F. (2006) Perilesional skin care. Fundaci6n

3M y Drug Farma, S.L., ISBN: 84-96724-03-4
Forrest R. D. (1982). Development of wound therapy from the Dark Ages
to the present. Journal of the Royal Society of Medicine, 75(4), 268-273.
https://doi.org/10.1177/014107688207500413

Hampton S. (2004). A guide to managing the surrounding skin of chronic,
exuding wounds. Professional nurse (London, England), 19(12), 30-32.
Jorge, S. A., & Dantas, S. (2004). Multiprofessional Approach to Wound
Care. Sao Paulo: Atheneu.

Moore PJ, Foster L. (2000). Cost benefits of two dressings in the
management of surgical wounds. Br J Nurs. Sep 28-Oct ;9(17):1128-32.
doi:10.12968/bjon.2000.9.17.5464.

Parreira, Ana; Marques, Rita (2017). Wounds - Manual of Good
Practices. Lidel. ISBN: 9789897520976.

Ramos, P.; Grilo, L.; Sousa, F.; Almeida, A.; Alves, P. (2021)
ABORDAGEM À

PEOPLE WITH SKIN INJURIES ASSOCIATED WITH HUMILITY.
Association Portuguese Wound Care. ISBN 978-989-54770-7-4
Voegeli D. (2008). The effect of washing and drying practices on skin
barrier function. Journal of wound, ostomy, and continence nursing:
official publication of The Wound, Ostomy and Continence Nurses

Society, 35(1), 84-90.
https://doi.org/10.1097/01.WON.0000308623.68582.d7

Yao, K., Bae, L., & Yew, W. P. (2013). Post-operative wound management. Australian family physician, 42(12), 867-870.

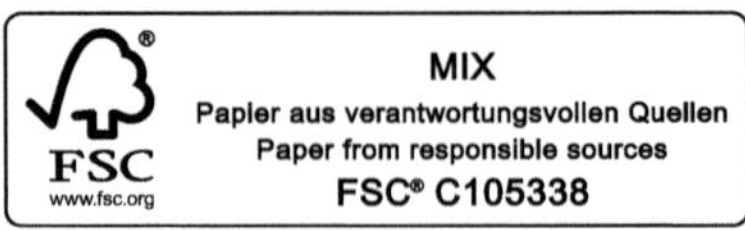

Printed by Books on Demand GmbH, Norderstedt / Germany